STAY IN THE GAME

5 Factors to Stay Employable as YOU Age

Debra Amandola, PhD

Page Solutions
541 Buttermilk Pike
Crescent Springs, KY 41017

Copyright © 2025 by Debra Amandola, PhD.

ISBN 979-8-89633-031-8 (softcover)
ISBN 979-8-89633-050-9 (hardcover)
ISBN 979-8-89633-047-9 (ebook)

All rights reserved. No part of this book may be reproduced or transmitted in any form or by any means, electronic or mechanical, including photocopying, recording, or by any information storage and retrieval system without express written permission from the author, except in the case of brief quotations embodied in critical reviews and certain other noncommercial uses permitted by copyright law.

This book is a work of fiction. Names, characters, places, and incidents are the product of the author's imagination or are used fictitiously. Any resemblance to actual locales, events, or persons, living or dead, is purely coincidental.

Printed in the United States of America.

DEDICATION

This book is dedicated to the thirteen women I interviewed for my dissertation research, each one inspiring. May they inspire others with their wisdom and dedication to working.

CONTENTS

Chapter 1—Introduction 7

Chapter 2—Enjoyment of Work 11

Chapter 3—Physical Health and Mental Sharpness 17

Chapter 4—Personal Resilience 21

Chapter 5—Work Relationships 27

Chapter 6—Continuous Learning / Relevant Deep Expertise 35

Chapter 7—Summary 39

Appendix 41

References by Chapter 43

Epilogue 47

CHAPTER 1

Introduction

I am writing this book, dear sisters, because many of us love the work we are doing and don't see our lives without it. In fact, we can learn from many of our sisters how to prevent not working. Yet, as people age, many are choosing to extend their working life if they can. The extended lifespan is now over 80 years old, and delaying retirement is appealing to many individuals based on numerous factors. Work, especially for those past retirement age, provides greater financial security, better health and vitality, and the ability to express a person's passion, which aids the individual in remaining active, engaged, and productive.

This book provides valuable information and insight for women of a variety of ages. Baby Boomers, who are wrestling with the decision to stay employed or retire, will find this material particularly useful so they can make the best, informed decision for their needs. Women who are Generation Xer's may also begin thinking and planning to prolong their career until age 70 or beyond. Additionally, the information in this book may appeal to Millennials as they explore their options and future in a career that they are passionate about.

The information and research in this book is based on my Doctoral Dissertation, which was completed in May, 2018. The qualitative study involved 13 women who were involved in active work from the ages of 66 – 100 and was collected in 2016. I will tell you many of their stories and a few of mine to help you. The themes that emerged are reflected in the chapters of this book. These themes are not quantifiable yet based on a qualitative research study with members of the population not in its entirety yet provides insight to support and prepare women as we age.

The book is organized to help readers reflect on each theme, which includes: meaning of work, physical health and mental sharpness, personal resilience, work relationships and continuous learning / deep relevant skills. In each chapter, there is an opportunity to complete self-assessments, and set direction for yourself and your needs. Use this as a workbook to help you be inspired and encouraged. I wanted to bring this material to you to help you to continue to work if you so choose to do this.

The following page, 5, in this book, is there to help you process your learnings and discoveries as you work through each chapter included in the book. Each chapter provides questions for you to consider for your specific circumstances and life. This is an interactive book and one that you could enjoy and find valuable. As you complete the questions in each chapter, the chapter questions will ask you to refer to page 5 to add your reflections from the specific questions. Once you have completed each section, you will have the notes to capture your learning and discovery so you can begin to do the things you want to do.

Please, have fun while you are reading and working through the materials in this book. Your relaxation will support you in being safe, honest, and helpful to yourself. There is no best answer. Your answer is the best answer!

Notes Page for Exercises by Chapter

Chapter	Reflection Questions
Chapter 2 – Enjoyment of Work	What are you committing to, in order to demonstrate enjoyment / passion for work, and how to stand out?
Chapter 3 – Physical Health & Mental Sharpness	What will you start, stop, and continue to do for physical health and mental sharpness?
Chapter 4 – Personal Resilience	What have you learned about personal resilience? What is your plan to enhance yours?
Chapter 5 – Work Relationships	What will you do to maximize your work relationships' effectiveness?
Chapter 6 – Continuous Learning & Relevant Deep Expertise	What are your commitments to continue learning and enhancing your expertise?
Chapter 7 – Summary	What is my overall learning from this material? What is going well? What do I need to enhance?

CHAPTER 2

Enjoyment of Work

Work is not appealing or enjoyable if it is boring, or something you do not like or feel skilled to do. This might be the job you can't wait to retire from and are counting the days until you can walk away. Depending on your age, however, leaving this position may not be in your best interest. Sass (2016) suggests your current employer provides the best possibility to stay employed beyond age 65 with greater financial rewards. However, if you do not enjoy your work, then you might need to reassess your current situation. A long-term friend of mine announced she is retiring in one week, counting the days. Juxtaposed to my position, I have a longing for a full-time, permanent position where I can have fun doing what I love.

You may love work because you love what you do, and the contribution you make to the organization in this position. All of the women interviewed for my dissertation, loved the work they each were involved and the organizations they did the work for and they made a strong contribution. An example of this is the college professor who loves to teach children to read and now she teaches teachers how to teach children to read. Another woman reported her ability to stay until beyond age 70 was to constantly ask herself and take action on "What can I do to make me indispensible in this organization?" This chapter will cover how to identify and find work that matches your values and passions. It will also help you identify your professional identity, as well as ways to find the work you love. Let's get started.

Values and Passions

Values and passions are a good place to start, as they function in together. They can both fuel and act as a motivator by informing your position in your career. Values are defined as factors that are most important to you, such as spirituality, health, achievement, integrity, and family happiness. They may change as you age. For example, as a younger woman, my personal values greatly influenced my perception of family happiness. Focusing on supporting the positive growth and development of my children and watching them develop into happy and capable adults is how I defined family happiness. Now that my children are adults, the focus of this value has shifted, and is more about creating fond memories with them, and enjoying and encouraging my grandchildren. It is imperative, however, that you understand each person is different and their respective values, and influences, will change and grow depending on each unique person. In the appendix, you will find a list of values. Please select the top 5 – 8 values for yourself (page 30). Once you identify them, it is valuable to write a statement about what this value means to you. You can add them to the first question on page 9.

Passion also influences your motivation levels and the drive inspiring you to push forward. Passions are defined as what you love and feel you have a calling to do. They can be affected by several aspects of your life, such as your personality, interests, goals, and your parents' occupations / business life. For example, my childhood was focused on family and friends were some of these people who came to stay at the resort my family owned and operated on a major lake. From my familial experiences, an avid interest in people surfaced. I changed my college major from medical technology to education. The goal was not to be a teacher, yet the field led me to helping individuals who were challenged emotionally, mentally, or physically. This grew into a career as counselor/ coach for working people. As this career progressed, exposure to leading outplacement seminars introduced me to work that was in line with my interests and motivations, and therefore, my passions: corporate training and organization development. This has been the focus of my career for many years. In contrast, a person who likes to take things apart as a child ended could end up with a career in biomedical electronics and repair imaging equipment. Passions can lead to natural progressions as we learn what we love and follow the path that motivates us the most.

Your passions may not be easily identifiable in the beginning of our career. They can become clearer as we age and gain more experience and perspective. Because of this, many people change careers midstream. This process has been described as climbing the ladder of success and realizing your ladder is on the wrong wall. A good example of this is a woman who prepared herself to work in corporate finance and ended up fulfilling a variety of roles in this field. During a 'managing your career' class she discovered she wanted to work with people exclusively. She discovered her manager was not willing to support her decision, which led to a series of life and career changes. This woman eventually married and relocated to another part of the United States, where several years later she had a Ph.D. in adult education and was working in an established career as a consultant in organization development. This woman eventually became an executive in a human resources position, which is exactly where she wanted to be. She followed her passions and chose to let those motivate her in the direction she wanted, despite obstacles saying otherwise.

One of the factors helping women to stay employable as they age is the energy and passion they show for the work each is involved with for their respective employer. The woman who is striving to be of vital importance used her unique skills, knowledge and abilities to do this. As a lawyer, she became the legal voice in the organization as well as use her Spanish bi-lingual ability to teach ethics courses in Latin speaking countries. This helped the organization to reach its business goals of expanding to Latin speaking countries. This can come across as motivation and enthusiasm in the workplace. This passion can also come from the interests and values each person holds. There are several questions to help you understand your passion and values.

Chapter 2 Reflections

Which values surfaced to be your top 5 -8?

What work do you feel passionate about?

What can you do to become vitally important to your organization?

On a scale of 1–10 (10 high), how would you rate your passion for this work?

What do you enjoy about this work?

How is this passion and enjoyment reflected in your behavior?

Please turn to page 5 to make notes about what you learned regarding your values, passions, and work meaning.

CHAPTER 3

Physical Health and Mental Sharpness

Physical health and mental sharpness are very important factors when considering work beyond age 65. My godmother used to say, "when you have health, you have everything." Engaging work positively impacts people, helping them maintain healthier and happier lives (Calvo, 2013). Vaillant (2002) found, in a longitudinal study over a 50-year span, that a happy-well person lived longer with higher quality life, than a sad-sick person. Both work and health are beneficial to each other. Let's take a detailed look at both physical health and mental sharpness.

Physical health is the ability to physically do the work that is needed for the position / duties of work and your life. Working 40 or more hours per week can be physically demanding. However, if you have work that you love, that love can help to fuel the energy needed for the work.

Getting and maintaining health is an ongoing practice. It requires exercise and nutrition. Finding time for exercise can be a challenge for a busy person, which is why identifying an exercise activity you enjoy is critical. Exercise can include: dancing, walking, tennis, running, gardening, yoga, aerobics, or a myriad of fitness classes. I have continued to walk with my dogs for the last 30 years. They are my accountability partners, which ensures I stay active. I have also chosen strength training, interval training, and yoga to keep myself in top shape.

One question may be 'how make time for physical movement into my busy life?' Time management experts suggest setting weekly goals for yourself. I try to walk up to 12 miles a week when working full time. I accomplish this by walking two miles over two days during the workweek, and then I walk four miles twice over the weekend. This allows time for other activities during the week, such as going to professional meetings, working late, participating in activities with children. An additional time management technique is making meals ahead of time to make it easier on other, busier days. If I don't reach 12 miles, the world does not end. I adjust and do the best I can. Be forgiving of yourself, while maintaining realistic goals. Most importantly, use your willpower and self-motivation to make your goals achievable. When my daughter was young, I exercised so I would be vital and vibrant when she had children. I saw exercising as an investment in my future. Now that she is 25, I can run and keep up with her young son. Newton's law of inertia states that a body at rest stays at rest, and a body in motion stays in motion, so ask yourself—which one do I want? I knew for sure I wanted to be a body in motion. This motion helps me to be in impeccable shape at age 64, and to create my best life and future with my family, values, passions, and career.

Nutrition is a key factor in living a healthy lifestyle. We constantly have an influx of ever changing diet suggestions, such as minimizing highly processed foods that are loaded with carbohydrates and sugar. Some individuals are choosing vegetarianism or veganism, which eliminates animal products from their diets. Occasionally this can be a values-based decision. Certain people have to eliminate gluten or chose to eat gluten-free. Each body is different; and will react differently to foods that are unique to you. Some bodies need carbs, while others cannot process them. If you want to explore any one of these eating patterns, I encourage you to do research, speak with a health professional, and experiment with what works for your body. For example, I ate as a vegetarian for a period of time and found I needed more lean protein in my diet. I was experiencing body aches due to this. As I added fish and chicken back to my diet, the pain went away. In April, 2014, my doctor suggested I try to eat gluten-free and asked me to read the book, "Wheat Belly" by William Davis. I chose to eat this way for one year. I lost 20 pounds in the first year and brain fog disappeared. Also, I noticed my fingers hurt when I eat gluten. I continue to watch and be mindful of the gluten I do eat, and I am especially cognizant of somatic symptoms. Now, I try to minimize gluten at each meal. Planning in advance makes this doable. Consider, however, that this is what works specifically for *my* body and *my* schedule. Every person is different, and it is up to you to take your own health and nutrition to the level you want it to be. Determine what works for you over time and experiment. Take note of what does and does not work. It will help you develop an eating plan that will work for you as you move through your life.

Mental health is just as, if not more so, important as physical health. Your physical fitness and nutrition will directly impact your mental sharpness. Mental sharpness helps you solve problems, create new ideas, and maximize your contribution to your life and work. Of the 13 women in the qualitative study, eight have terminal degrees, and all of them earned these degrees over age 40. Calvo (2006) states that work can help you stay sharp, and the women interviewed in my study agreed. Reading, writing, traveling, listening, and engaging in work can support and maintain mental sharpness. All create a way to exercise your mind and mental acuity.

The Great American Read (PBS) has encouraged more people to read and become involved in book clubs. I participate in a book club that has broadened my normal reading scope, in addition to providing accountability for reading. Find activities you enjoy that will keep you mentally sharp, challenge your brain, awareness, and thinking.

Exercise, nutrition, and continually working on mental sharpness will positively impact your vitality both physically and mentally. Putting goals in place with weekly planning will help you create the life you want today and set you up for success in the future.

Chapter 3 Reflections

What are some of your plans for time management?

What are your plans for physical exercise in your life?

What would you like to do to enhance your nutritional plan?

What activities do you love that would help you with mental sharpness?

Turn to page 5 and make notes about your what your have learned, your goals, and commitments regarding your physical health and mental sharpness.

CHAPTER 4

Personal Resilience

Personal resilience and positive psychology are extremely important to thriving and living a full life as one ages. Personal resilience is defined as the ability to cope with adversity and positively adapt (Lavretsky & Irwin, 2007; Nash, 2011; Wagnild, 2003). Reivich and Shatte (2002) suggest resilience is essential to success and happiness. Wagnild (2003) proposes resilience has been correlated with many aspects of successful aging that include: life satisfaction, morale, stress management, lower levels of depression, better health, and health promoting behaviors. Obviously, personal resilience is key to being able to stay employed beyond age 65 and age well. Without resilience, an individual is unable to adapt in ever changing work places, as well as changes that occur throughout the lifespan process.

Positive psychology is defined as taking a growth and learning approach to life to continually improve as you go through life in other words, flourishing. Seligman (2002) while at the University of Pennsylvania started the field of studying why some people continue to flourish as they go about their life.

Klohnen, Vandewater, and Young (1996) found that ego-resilient individuals lived actively and were meaningfully involved in the world. These individuals that have achieved results with a variety of skills and personality traits. These skills and traits include a positive and energetic approach to life, mastery of functioning skills, perceptive and insightful, and interpersonally skilled to create warm and open relations with other people. This is indicative of both resilience and positive psychology. Positive psychology is influential for moving research among adults and older adults, and consistent with intra-individual flexibility and adaptability (Baltes, 1997; Bergman & Wallace, 1999). These traits allow a person, despite their age, to move forward in a fluid, and flexible manner.

As we age, obstacles tend to become more prevalent simply due to the aging process. The difficulties we face include multiple interpersonal or financial losses, losses of personal or familial health, or independence of self or family member. Losing a spouse or child during your life is substantially impactful at all levels and losing a valued work position or role can also negatively impact your life and challenge resilience. Being able to experience these adversities and positively adapt is extremely valuable and crucial to moving forward.

Polk (1997) synthesized 26 studies and created four organizing categories to provide a comprehensive approach to defining and improving resilience. These include:

- Dispositional Patterns (physical and psychological factors). These can best be described as the parts of you that are part of your being. An example of this is a woman I interviewed lost her father at age 17 and decided to stay and home and support her family, her husband died later in her life as well as her son. She describes herself as positive and her blood type supports this with a B+ type.

- Relational Patterns (social roles and relationships). A woman I interviewed created a positive relationship with each new leader she supported, even when the leader was perceived negatively by others. She leveraged this to be the most effective legal advisor to the organization and to create the opportunity to use her bi-lingual skills and teach ethics courses in Latin

American speaking countries. All of these made her important to the organization and her direct manager.

- Situational Pattern (how individuals face the world). One woman interviewed said her life exploded once she completed her PhD. She became a college professor and relocated to climb the academic career ladder and over time became the dean of the department by building the experience to catapult her to this level of responsibility. She loved living in a variety of locations and studying the diversity in locations such as West Virginia, Oregon, and south Florida. She loves taking her granddaughters to London or Paris for the holidays.
- Philosophical Pattern (Personal beliefs and values). One woman interviewed became a long-term executive in a telecommunications company and used her ability to get along with men (she had four brothers). She loved to make things better where ever she worked and did this for her entire career (something she learned as a babysitter at age 13.)

Now you can begin to identify ways to enhance your resilience with these patterns. The following questions relate to these patterns. Be honest with yourself.

Disposition is defined as a person's inherent qualities of mind and character. How would you describe your disposition?

Relational patterns are about how you relate to the people in your world. What patterns do you see in your life?

Situational patterns have to do with how you face the world. Do you see the world as cold and cruel, or warm and inviting? What would you say about how you have coped with situations and how have your skills increased in effectiveness over the years?

Philosophical patterns address your personal beliefs and values. What are your personal beliefs and values?

The women interviewed in my research had a dispositional pattern of happy and are able to deal with anything. They are optimistic and see the world as friendly. Vaillant (2002) found the happy / well individuals lived longer and high-quality lives than the sad/sick individuals. The woman interviewed have also formed relationships that are supportive and encouraging. Some of them have few friends and some had many friends, depending on their desire and time available. They have become more skilled with handling situational adversity, which for many of them, began early in life. Their skills improved as they were continually tested as their lives evolved. In the research, their philosophical pattern pointed to that of an awareness of a universal power for good, and the desire to do good in their lives.

Wagnild (1993) suggests five factors to maximize adaptability, which is crucial to true resilience. These five factors succinctly categorize perspective, and the impact differing perspectives can have on your life and your ability to adapt.

1. Equanimity: a balanced perspective of life.
2. Meaningfulness: a sense of purpose in life.
3. Perseverance: the ability to keep going despite setbacks.

4. Existential aloneness: the recognition of one's unique path and the acceptance of one's life.
5. Self-reliance: the belief in one's self and capabilities.

Personal resilience and positive psychology are interrelated concepts that impact your ability to age well. Enhancing your personal resilience will help you continue working as organizations are changing and evolving and challenging personal resilience as associates work within a respective organization. This resilience in you will help you say employable and looking at this in your life is excessively valuable.

Chapter 4 Reflections

What are the various roles you have in life, and what makes them meaningful?

What is your purpose in life?

Do you see something to the end when you want it? Don't want it?

What makes your path in life unique? What makes you unique?

What are your greatest capabilities?

What have you learned about personal resilience?

What are you willing to commit to when moving forward on your own personal resilience?

Please turn to page 5 and make notes about your personal resilience.

CHAPTER 5

Work Relationships

Work relationships are crucial in helping women maintain employment past standard retirement age. Social connections are important to meaningfulness; and contribute both personally and professionally to happiness. The women interviewed were very specific in characteristics that contributed to positive work relationships. They emphasized the importance of collaboration and had humility. Traits such as selfishness and ruthlessness were not a positive factor in work relationships, and something that should be avoided if you choose to extend your work life. Ross and Mirowsky (1995) propose that social interaction and support are important factors to staying employed. In this chapter, several types of social connections will be explored, including networking, teamwork, building allies at work, mentoring, building relationships across the organization, and learning partners. Social connections in the personal aspect of life are important also; and will be touched upon briefly. Several different kinds of work relationships will be the focus of this chapter. Included are manager relationships, networking, team building, allies, mentors and mentees, and friendships.

Conger & Church (2018) propose your direct manager in an organization has a huge impact on you, the employee, as you age. They know you, judge you, and represent you in the rest of the organization. If you think about helping your manager achieve their goals, it is linked to their rewards and advancements. Ways you can ensure you are capitalizing on this are to be sensitive and adapting with every manager you have, making your manager's significant tasks as your highest priority, performing everything you do as if you are at a higher level, demonstrating extreme initiative beyond the significant tasks, take things off your managers plate (preferable things you do well), and adapting and mirroring the style of your manager. Paying attention to this relationship is an extremely important relationship to care for and nurture.

Networking is the process of building relationships outside of your specific organization. You can do internal networking life the woman who had lunch with customers. You can also do external networking. This can occur through professional organizations such as Society of Human Resources (SHRM), or other professional organizations that are part of your specific profession. These connections can help you in a number of different ways, such as learning partners for benchmarking and idea creation. They also help others get to know you outside of your direct organization. If you work in a part of an organization that keeps you isolated, networking will also help you meet others within the organization itself. For example, one of the women interviewed had lunch with a department head every day, as these are her customers. The more details she knows about what they need, the more she is able to deliver high-value customer information.

Team building includes working with a group toward a common goal. Two of the women interviewed talked about collaborating with their respective team to create valuable products for their customer base. It was teamwork that created the amazing products, because several of them worked together in the creation process. Personally, I have found I prefer to be an internal consultant rather than an external consultant, primarily because I like to work with other people in the organization toward a common purpose. Collaboration not only allows for new ideas and products, but also allows for work relationships to be established and maintained.

Building allies at work is another factor in creating strong social contacts that will help you stay employed. Doing so with your direct manager team is a valuable method. The woman who had lunch with different department heads over the course of the year is creating allies by understanding their needs so she is able to provide high value service. As in other influential factors, this process can be planned and tailored to meet your needs and schedule. Try to set a goal to meet one or two new people per month; and commit to building and strengthening a relationship with them. It is also valuable to create a board of directors (3 -5) for you in your career. These individuals would encourage and provide ideas to you as you move through your life. A Board of Directors is a steering committee for you in your career and can help you for several years. You might select people for your board that represent skills or perspectives you don't have. You also may want members who are upbeat and positive and can help you with encouragement and support you with honest and kind ways. You can ask them for monthly, quarterly or annual meetings.

Mentoring is a different kind of relationship. This is a person who can advise you, promote you, advocate for you, and/ or provide a sounding board. You can also be a mentor and learn from your mentee. The mentor often learns more than the mentee. The mentee drives the relationship and the meetings, while the mentor learns from all of this activity. This also appeals to the shift that occurs as we age with the increased desire to leave a legacy or share expertise, as well as keeping older workers up to date with new information the younger generation is bringing in.

Building relationships across the organization is different than building allies. Workers have reported that they are able to accomplish tasks and projects because they know people across their organization. This process occurs over time if you take the opportunity to establish relationships with a variety of people within your organization. Chances for this will occur naturally through seeking help from other departments or team projects that may be cross-functional. Relationship building within an organization is also possible when the organization does service work in the community, such as Habitat for Humanity, March of Dimes, etc.

Learning partners can include those individuals you meet through challenging work, developing new products, and participation in leadership development programs. These partnerships can offer valuable insights and new approaches. You can also share insights that are useful and valuable to the other person.

An additional method that can affect your work relationships is the Law of Reciprocity. This leverages the idea that when you do something for someone else, they feel it is important to do something for you. In short, they will reciprocate your action. For this to occur, you must make an offer to an associate, which could include anything task related, or even something more personal in nature. If this is something you can easily do and would be considered of high value for the other person, it may well be accepted. You can also accept the offer of another.

The Law of Reciprocity can also be used for personal social connections, which can be extremely valuable and worth investing in over your lifetime. The categories of these social connections include family, friends, and neighbors. As an example, several years ago, I was on my homeowners' association board of directors. I received a medical report on my mom's brain after she died and I did not understand it. One of my peers was the director of pharmacology at a local hospital and he interpreted the report for me. This was incredibly helpful and valuable to me at this point in time. Recently, a good friend and I were attending graduate school together. We committed to participate in each other's graduation and it was extremely meaningful to both of us.

Below are two drawings I suggest you use to "inventory" your social and work connections. Please write the names of the people who meet the varied criteria. The inner circle includes your most trusted and intimate connections. As you move out of the circle, less closeness and intimacy are shared yet a relationship exists. When examining your circle, what movement in these connections would you like to make in the coming years? With this exercise you can also see areas that need attention. You might also need to add what kind of connection you have with each person. This may help you to identify areas of improvement.

Debra Amandola, PhD

Work Connection Map

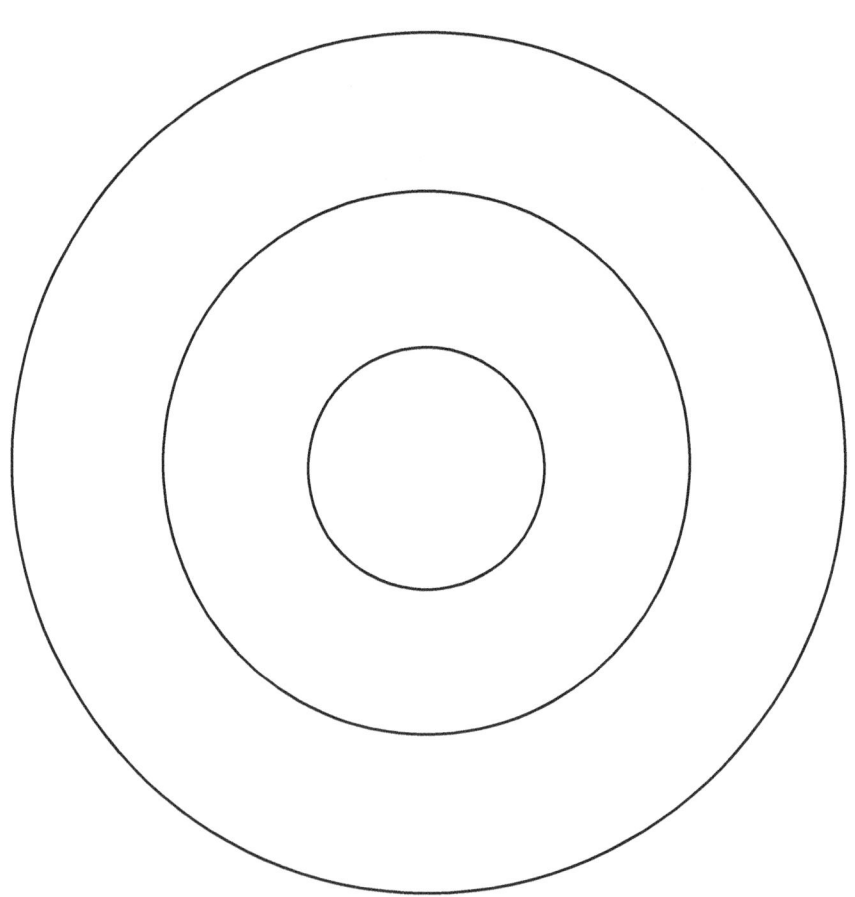

Stay in the GAME

Social Connection Map

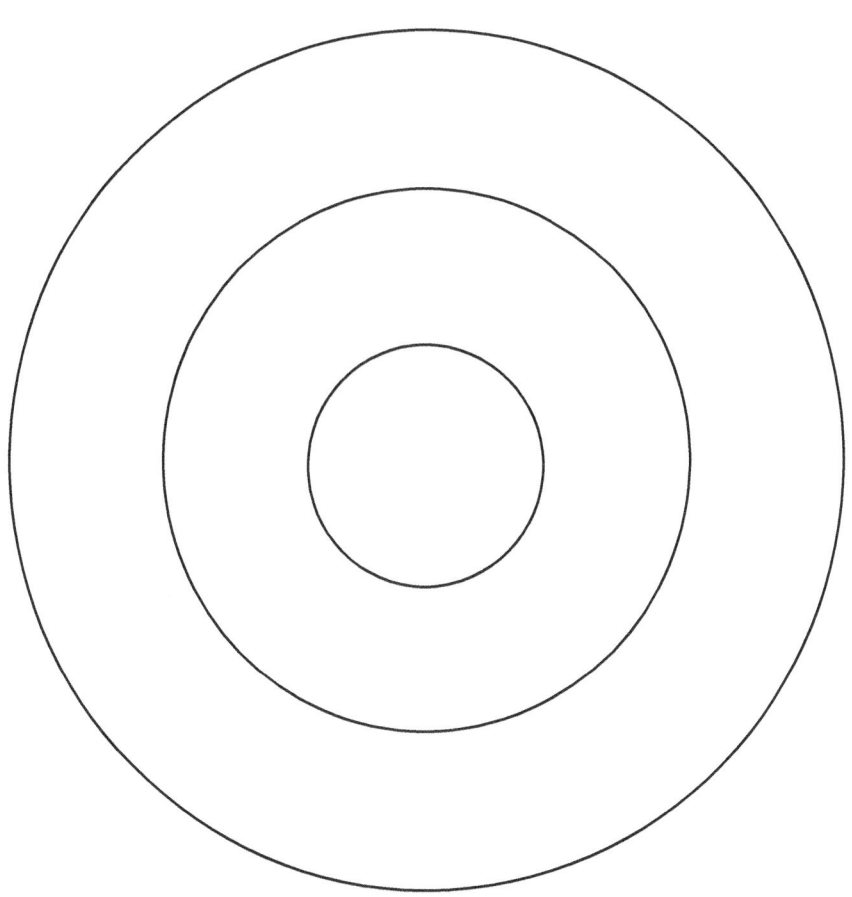

Chapter 5 Reflections

What movements are you going to focus on in your work and social connections?

What do you want to increase?

What do you want to decrease?

Please turn to page 5 and make notes about your learning and commitments on work relationships.

CHAPTER 6

Continuous Learning / Relevant Deep Expertise

Keeping skills current and relevant to employer and company needs is important to staying employed. The challenge many of us may run into is that some of our best skills have become part of our personality, also called the unconscious competent person. This is a person who has developed skills and done them for so long, it is difficult to see these talents as skills. What was once considered a skill is now an intrinsic part of our personality, and sometimes a habit we are unaware of. Lifelong learning is defined as an individual who continues to learn their entire life. College learning is one way to do this as well as learning new ways to do things or learning new things to support automation of functions as work processes evolve with technology.

Many of the women interviewed had lifelong learning. This is demonstrated as eight of the 13 interviewed had advanced degrees that were achieved after age 40. Since most of the women have worked in the same area for their career, they had deep expertise. Many of the eight who earned degrees talked about how their life changed for the better once their desired educational level was attained. Additionally, the women looked at the direction of the organization's goals, enabling them to think about the contribution they wanted to make to meet the organization's evolving needs. This helped each woman stay relevant and valuable in her career field. Many said work helped them keep their skills current and evolving based on the duties and responsibilities the position included.

Deep relevant skills and those skills that an individual has mastered. At times they have become part of the uniqueness of the person this individual has become over their entire life. Two examples from the women interviewed surface. First, the woman is now a college professor now teaching teachers how to teach reading to children. She mentioned in the interview she read to her children voraciously and believes strongly in children learning to read. This is her brand something she knows well. The second person became a lawyer after the age of 40 and easily passed the bar exam. She is now provided legal advice to her employer as well as teaching ethics courses to students in America and in Latin America. She can do this because she is bi-lingual. Both legal areas and the bi-lingual are interests and her language skills have been with her most of her life. I want to share one caution to you. In 2018, I left my previous employer and was unable to find a new position because I was over-qualified, an experienced person with a PhD. This was a harsh reality to me. I have reflected, would I change getting my PhD? I have said no. Some of my professional friends have suggested I take it off my resume. Yet, it will allow me do what I am doing with this book and leading retreats for women.

The desire to continue to be a life-long learner and have found areas that have interested them for many years with the time to hone the skills for the area have created deep relevant skills.

You will now have the chance to look at your own learning and skills and see how they fit with this factor. Turn to the next page.

Chapter 6 Reflections

What has been the direction of your career so far?

What are you dreaming of doing?

What have you done to update your education or learning?

What have been your most recent / memorable accomplishments?

Taking each accomplishment into consideration, what are your greatest and most satisfying skills?

Turn to page 5 and make notes about what you have learned regarding continuous learning and demonstrating relevant and deep expertise.

Notes for Skills Analysis

CHAPTER 7

Summary

This book has taken you through the five factors that influenced and supported many women who choose to remain employed beyond age 65., in other words they are staying in the game. By completing the exercises in each chapter and then adding your reflections on page 5, you have set the foundation and created a plan to stay in the game beyond the typical retirement age and delay retirement. The areas covered include keeping your passion and energy high and motivated for the work you love, keeping your physical and mental abilities sharp, using resilience to stay positive and motivated, building work relationships to support you at work as well as your social relationships that support staying in the game, and keeping your skills and develop deep expertise sharp. You can find your reflections on page 5 that personalizes this vital information for you.

Considering many individuals retire, get bored, and re-enter the workforce, I suggest you stick with your main career until you are sure you want to retire and have carefully considered your plan and goals. Each individual is unique, with a unique sense of purpose and lifelong goals. Evaluate your values and passions, determine what you need your life to be, and carefully decide what is right for you. I sincerely hope you have enjoyed this journey of self-discovery.

I welcome your comments and questions. Please feel free to contact me at amandoladeb@gmail.com.

This project is a passion of mine, as it effects my decision to extend my career and understand the factors that contribute to this decision. I, myself, am aiming to work until age 70 or beyond because I love the work I do. I was unable to be employed because I was over qualified in my market at age 64. I completed my Ph.D. at age 63. My chosen profession is corporate training and development, specifically leadership and career development. I have chosen to take my life in a different direction by writing this book, designing retreats for women, and doing adjunct professor work in local colleges and universities. I live in the Midwest with my husband of 39 years, have 3 dogs, and stay in good physical shape. Our children live locally, aged 34 and 25, and they are both married. We have two grandsons, who we love to be active with. I love the Lake of the Ozarks and snow skiing.

APPENDIX

Below is a list of twenty-five values laid out in a block fashion. Place a large X in the block that contains a value you can live without. Continue to cross out values until you have 10 that you are important to you. Then search your soul and leave only five unmarked, these will be your top most important values.

Acheivement	Adventure	Affection	Approval	Challenge
Competition	Family	Freedom	Health	Financial Security
Independence	Integrity	Loyalty	Order	Relationships
Recognition	Prestige	Power	Security	Self-Acceptance
Spiritual	Wealth	Wisdom	Pleasure	Self-Development

    The alignment of these values significantly impact your decisions and your behavior.

What are your top 5 values?

_____
_____
_____
_____
_____

REFERENCES BY CHAPTER

Chapter Two – Enjoyment of Work

Conger, J.A. & Church, A.H. (2018). *The high potential's advantage: Get noticed, impress your bosses, and become a top leader.* Boston, MA. Harvard Business Review Press Press.

Haley, Ivy. (1996) *Discovering your purpose.* Mission, KS: SkillPath Publications.

Sass, S. (2016). How do non-financial factors affect retirement decisions? *Center For Retirement Research at Boston College, 16,* 1 – 5.

Chapter Three – Physical Health and Mental Sharpness

Calvo, E. (2006). Does working longer make people healthier and happier? *An issue in brief: Center for Retirement Research at Boston College, 2,* 1 – 9.

Calvo, E. Sarkisian, N., & Tamborini, C.R. (2013). Casual effects of retirement timing on subjective physical and emotional health. *Journal of Gerontology Series B: Psychological Sciences and Social Sciences, 68,* 73 – 84.

Vaillant, G.E. (2002). *Aging well: surprising guideposts to a happier life from the landmark Harvard study of adult development.* Boston, MA: Little Brown & Company.

Chapter 4 – Personal Resilience

Baltes, P.B. (1997). On the incomplete architecture of human ontogeny: Selection, optimization, and a compensation as foundation of development theory. *American Psychologist, 52,* 266 – 380.

Bergman, C.S., & Wallace, K.A. (1999). Resiliency in later life. In T.L. Whitman, T.V.

Merluzzi & R.D. White(Eds.) *Life span perspectives on health and illness* (pp. 207 – 227). Hllsdale, NJ: Lawrence Erlbaum Associates.

Klohnen, E.C., Vandewater, E.A., & Young, A. (1996). Negotiating the middle years: Ego resiliency and successful midlife adjustment in women. *Psychology and Aging, 11,* 431 – 442.

Lavertsky, H., & Irwin, M.R. (2007). Resilience and aging. *Aging Health, 3,* 309 – 323.

Nash, K. (2001, September 21). *Personnel resilience. St. Louis Business Journal,* 63A.

Polk, L.V. (1997). Toward a middle-range theory of resilience. *Advances in Nursing, 19,* 1 – 13.

Reivich, K., & Shatte, A. (2002). *The resiience factor: 7 essential skills for overcoming life's obstacles.* New York, NY: Random House.

Seligman, M. (2002). Authentic Happiness. New York, NY: Simon & Schuster.

Wagnild, G. (2003). Resilience and successful aging: Comparison among low and high income older adults. *Journal of Gerontological Nursing, 29,* 42 – 49.

Wagnild, G., & Young, H.M. (1993). Development and psychometric evaluation of the Resilience Scale. *Journal of Nursing, 1,* 165 – 177.

Chapter Five – Work Relationships

Ross, C.E., & Mirowsky, J. (1995). Does employment effect health? *Journal of Health And Social Behavior, 36,* 236 – 243.

NOTES PAGE

EPILOGUE

Since my dissertation was complete in 2018, my interest in this area has continued. I have continued to talk with many people, men and women and all have said they are interested in this topic. After I left Garmin in 2018, I found discrimination in the world for full time, permanent employment at age of 64 with 35 years of experience and a PhD. A few years later, I applied for the position of a leadership coach for Lee Hecht Harrison and have been doing this since 2021. My husband, a field service engineer, with GE Health continues to work at age 71.

Many people have told me they. Also want to work beyond the retirement age of 66 for a number of reasons and love learning what they can do to ensure this is a reality. Also, younger people have been interested to ensure they have the ability to work as long as they want.

My Father, worked until he was 82. It was as an apartment owner and part time, yet he loved the work and it gave him pleasure.

www.ingramcontent.com/pod-product-compliance
Lightning Source LLC
Chambersburg PA
CBHW030307030426
42337CB00012B/622